EXERCISES FOR PARKINSON'S DISEASE

Effective Exercises For Beginners And Seniors To Manage Symptoms And Improve Quality Of Life

Christina J. Whitley

Table of contents

INTRODUCTION

In the world of health management, where every move can feel like a battle against a body in turmoil, there exists a guide offering a glimpse of hope and vitality, a guide for exercises tailored to those with Parkinson's disease. Let me introduce you to the vibrant stories that unfold within these exercises.

Imagine Sarah, a once lively individual whose laughter used to fill every room. But when Parkinson's entered her life, it overshadowed her joy with daily challenges. Tasks became struggles, and even walking turned into a careful dance with uncertainty.

Then, she discovered this guide—a collection of exercises designed specifically for those navigating Parkinson's. With a mix of skepticism and hope, Sarah began this journey. Little did she know how deeply it would impact her life.

As she engaged in gentle stretches, Sarah felt a release from the stiffness Parkinson's had imposed. Each stretch became a small triumph, gradually restoring her body's flexibility and freedom of movement.

But the guide didn't just benefit her physically. It empowered her to understand her symptoms and regain control. Balance training gave her confidence, correcting her posture both physically and spiritually.

Through muscle strengthening routines and cardiovascular workouts, Sarah found newfound strength. The exercises became not just physical movements but a testament to her resilience and endurance.

As she delved into hand-eye coordination drills, Sarah rediscovered the artistry in her movements. Each exercise was a celebration of coordination, a testament to the precision her body could still achieve.

Vocal and swallowing exercises became a gateway to expression and nourishment. They helped Sarah defy the challenges of Parkinson's, allowing her to express herself and eat safely.

This guide isn't just a compilation of exercises; it's a saga of triumphs, big and small. It's a journey of reclaiming agency, fostering community, and embracing the interconnectedness of physical and emotional well-being.

Join us on this journey through the guide to exercises for Parkinson's, a path illuminated with hope, vitality, and purpose. Together, let's paint a canvas of resilience and possibility with every exercise, a canvas waiting to be colored by hope and joy. Welcome to a narrative of movement, a story where every step signifies strength and vitality.

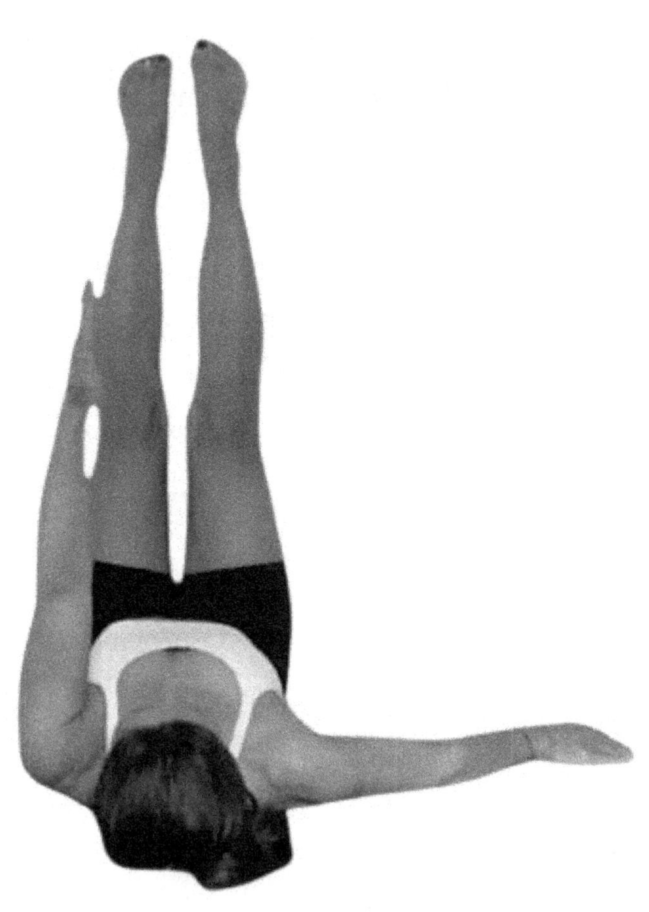

CHAPTER 1

Understanding Parkinson's Symptoms

Parkinson's disease is a complex neurodegenerative disorder that significantly impacts a person's motor functions and, in many cases, their overall quality of life. A comprehensive understanding of the symptoms associated with Parkinson's is essential for early diagnosis, effective management, and improved patient outcomes.

The hallmark symptoms of Parkinson's disease often become apparent gradually, making it important for individuals and healthcare professionals to be vigilant. One of the primary manifestations is tremors, involuntary rhythmic shaking that commonly occurs in the hands, fingers, or other extremities, particularly when at rest. These tremors can be subtle initially but tend to progress over time, affecting daily activities such as writing, eating, or handling objects.

Bradykinesia, or slowed movement, is another key symptom of Parkinson's. Individuals may notice a gradual reduction in their ability to initiate and complete physical movements. Simple tasks, like getting up from a chair or turning over in bed, become more challenging. Bradykinesia can lead to a general feeling of stiffness and may result in a shuffling gait as the disease advances.

Rigidity is characterized by increased resistance in the muscles, contributing to stiffness and a limited range of motion. This stiffness can be particularly pronounced in the arms, legs, and neck. Rigidity often makes it difficult for individuals with Parkinson's to perform fluid, coordinated movements.

Perhaps one of the most concerning symptoms is postural instability, where individuals experience difficulty maintaining balance. This instability can lead to an increased risk of falls, posing significant safety concerns for those living with Parkinson's. Addressing postural instability is crucial for maintaining independence and preventing injuries.

Beyond these primary motor symptoms, Parkinson's can manifest in various non-motor symptoms, further complicating the clinical picture. These may include:

- **Cognitive Changes:** Some individuals with Parkinson's experience cognitive decline, including difficulties with memory, attention, and executive function.

- **Autonomic Dysfunction:** Parkinson's can affect the autonomic nervous system, leading to issues such as blood pressure fluctuations, sweating abnormalities, and digestive problems.

- **Sleep Disturbances:** Many individuals with Parkinson's struggle with sleep disturbances, including insomnia, restless legs, and frequent waking during the night.

Understanding these diverse symptoms allows healthcare professionals to make a comprehensive diagnosis and tailor treatment plans to address the specific challenges faced by each individual. Moreover, it empowers individuals and their families to recognize changes early on, fostering proactive management strategies.

Diagnosing Parkinson's is often a clinical process, relying on a thorough examination of medical history, symptom presentation, and, in some cases, specialized imaging studies. It's important to note that there is no single definitive test for Parkinson's disease, making the expertise of neurologists and movement disorder specialists critical in the diagnostic process.

In conclusion, a nuanced understanding of Parkinson's symptoms is vital for early detection and effective management. By recognizing the diverse ways in which the disease manifests, healthcare professionals and individuals alike can work collaboratively to optimize care, improve quality of life, and enhance the overall well-being of those living with Parkinson's disease.

Benefits of Exercise for Parkinson's

1. Improved Mobility: Regular exercise, including stretching and aerobic activities, helps combat the stiffness and rigidity associated with Parkinson's disease, promoting better mobility and flexibility.

2. Enhanced Balance and Stability: Targeted exercises focusing on balance and coordination contribute to increased stability, reducing the risk of falls and improving overall postural control.

3. Strengthened Muscles: Muscle strength tends to decline in individuals with Parkinson's, impacting daily activities. Resistance training and weight-bearing exercises can help maintain and build muscle strength, supporting functional independence.

4. Fine-Tuned Motor Skills: Purposeful and repetitive movements in exercise routines contribute to the preservation and improvement of motor skills, aiding in tasks that require precision and coordination.

5. Mood Elevation: Exercise stimulates the release of endorphins, the body's natural mood enhancers. This can help alleviate symptoms of depression and anxiety that often accompany Parkinson's disease.

6. Cognitive Benefits: Emerging research suggests that regular physical activity may have cognitive benefits for individuals with Parkinson's, potentially slowing down cognitive decline and supporting overall brain health.

7. Cardiovascular Health: Engaging in aerobic exercises, such as walking, cycling, or swimming, contributes to improved cardiovascular health. This is especially important as individuals with Parkinson's may be at a higher risk of cardiovascular issues.

8. Social Interaction: Group exercise classes or activities provide an opportunity for social engagement, reducing feelings of isolation and fostering a sense of community among individuals living with Parkinson's and their caregivers.

9. Stress Reduction: Exercise is a powerful stress reliever, helping individuals manage the emotional and psychological challenges associated with Parkinson's disease. Techniques such as yoga and tai chi can be particularly beneficial.

10. Better Sleep: Regular physical activity can positively impact sleep patterns, addressing common sleep disturbances experienced by individuals with Parkinson's. Improved sleep contributes to overall well-being and quality of life.

Incorporating a well-rounded exercise program tailored to individual abilities and preferences can significantly enhance the overall health and well-being of individuals with Parkinson's disease. It not only addresses the physical challenges associated with the condition but also promotes emotional resilience and an improved quality of life. Always consult with healthcare professionals to design a safe and effective exercise plan based on individual needs and capabilities.

CHAPTER 2

Warm-Up and Mobility

Gentle Stretches for Flexibility:

1. Neck Stretch:

- Sit or stand comfortably.
- Slowly tilt your head to one side, bringing your ear toward your shoulder.
- Hold for 15-30 seconds, feeling a gentle stretch along the side of your neck.
- Repeat on the other side.

2. Shoulder Blade Stretch:

- Sit or stand with a straight back.
- Bring your right arm across your chest.

- Use your left hand to gently pull your right arm closer to your chest, feeling a stretch in your shoulder blade.

- Hold for 15-30 seconds and switch sides.

3. Seated Forward Bend:

- Sit on the floor with your legs extended in front of you.

- Slowly hinge at your hips and reach forward toward your toes.

- Keep your back straight and feel the stretch along your hamstrings and lower back.

- Hold for 20-30 seconds, breathing deeply.

Range of Motion Exercises:

1. Shoulder Circles:

- Stand with your feet shoulder-width apart.

- Slowly lift your shoulders toward your ears, then roll them back and down in a circular motion.

- Repeat for 10-15 repetitions and then reverse the direction.

2. Ankle Alphabet:

- Sit on a chair with your feet lifted off the ground.

- Imagine you're writing the alphabet with your toes, moving your ankles in a controlled and deliberate manner.

- This exercise promotes flexibility in the ankles and helps improve range of motion.

3. Hip Flexor Stretch:

- Stand with your feet hip-width apart.

- Take a step forward with your right foot into a lunge position.

- Lower your hips toward the floor, feeling a stretch in the front of your left hip.

- Hold for 15-30 seconds, then switch legs.

These exercises for gentle stretches and range of motion are designed to promote flexibility, alleviate stiffness, and enhance overall joint mobility. Always perform exercises within your comfort range and consult with a healthcare professional if you have any concerns or specific conditions.

CHAPTER 3

Balance and Posture Improvement

Balance Training for Stability:

1. Single Leg Stand:

- Stand near a sturdy surface for support.

- Lift one foot off the ground and balance on the other.

- Hold for 10-30 seconds, gradually increasing the time as your balance improves.

- Switch legs and repeat.

2. Heel-to-Toe Walk:

- Position the heel of one foot directly in front of the toes of the opposite foot.

- Walk forward in a straight line, placing the heel of each foot directly in front of the toes of the other foot.

- Focus on a fixed point ahead to help maintain balance.

- Perform for 10-15 steps.

3. Balance Ball Exercises:

- Stand with feet hip-width apart, holding a small balance ball.

- Lift one foot off the ground and balance on the other while holding the ball.

- Gradually introduce small movements, such as lifting the ball overhead.

- Switch legs and repeat.

Posture Correction Exercises:

1. Wall Angels:

- Stand with your back against a wall.

- Lift your arms to shoulder height, bending elbows at 90 degrees.

- Slowly slide arms up the wall, then back down, maintaining contact with the wall.

- This exercise helps improve shoulder and upper back posture.

2. Chin Tucks:

- Sit or stand with a straight back.

- Gently tuck your chin toward your chest, keeping your eyes forward.

- Hold for a few seconds, feeling a stretch in the neck and upper back.

- Repeat for 10-15 repetitions.

3. Plank with Shoulder Blade Squeeze:

- Start in a plank position, maintaining a straight line from head to heels.

- Squeeze your shoulder blades together without arching your back.

- Hold for 10-15 seconds, then relax.

- This exercise strengthens core muscles and promotes proper spinal alignment.

These balance training and posture correction exercises are designed to enhance stability, improve balance, and promote better alignment. Incorporate them into your routine gradually, ensuring proper form and consulting with a healthcare professional if you have specific concerns or conditions.

CHAPTER 4

Strength and Endurance Building

Muscle Strengthening Routines:

1. Bodyweight Squats:

- Stand with feet shoulder-width apart.

- Lower your body as if sitting back into a chair, keeping your back straight.

- Engage your leg muscles and return to the starting position.

- Repeat for 12-15 repetitions.

2. Bent-Over Rows:

- Hold a dumbbell in each hand, palms facing your body.

- Bend at the hips, keeping your back straight, and let your arms hang down.

- Lift the weights towards your chest, squeezing your shoulder blades.

- Lower the weights back down and repeat for 10-12 repetitions.

3. Lunges:

- Take a step forward with your right foot, lowering your body until both knees are bent at a 90-degree angle.

- Push off with your right foot to return to the starting position.

- Repeat with the left foot.

- Perform 10-12 lunges on each leg.

Cardiovascular and Aerobic Workouts:

1. Brisk Walking or Jogging:

- Engage in brisk walking or light jogging, depending on your fitness level.

- Aim for at least 30 minutes, gradually increasing intensity and duration over time.

- This simple yet effective cardiovascular exercise enhances heart health and overall fitness.

2. Cycling:

- Whether on a stationary bike or outdoors, cycling is an excellent aerobic workout.

- Start with a moderate pace and increase intensity as you build endurance.

- Aim for 20-30 minutes of continuous cycling.

3. Jumping Jacks:

- Stand with feet together and arms at your sides.

- Jump while spreading your legs and raising your arms overhead.

- Return to the starting position with another jump.

- Incorporate jumping jacks into your routine for 5-10 minutes as a high-intensity aerobic option.

These muscle strengthening routines and cardiovascular workouts contribute to overall physical health and well-being. Always start with an appropriate level of intensity and consult with a healthcare professional before beginning a new exercise regimen, especially if you have any existing health concerns.

CHAPTER 5

Co-ordination and Motor Skills

Hand-Eye Coordination Drills:

1. Ball Toss and Catch:

- Stand facing a partner or a wall.

- Toss a small ball back and forth, focusing on accuracy and catching with one hand.

- Gradually increase the distance and speed to challenge hand-eye coordination.

2. Juggling Scarves:

- Begin with lightweight scarves or soft objects.

- Toss one scarf into the air, and as it descends, toss another.

- Practice gradually incorporating more scarves to enhance coordination skills.

3. Reaction Ball Bouncing:

- Use a reaction ball, which bounces unpredictably.
- Stand a short distance away and bounce the ball.
- Try to catch the ball as it rebounds in different directions, improving reflexes and coordination.

Fine Motor Skill Exercises:

1. Finger Tapping:

- Tap each fingertip to your thumb in a coordinated and rhythmic manner.
  - Start slowly and gradually increase the speed.
  - This exercise enhances finger dexterity and control.

2. Pick-Up Sticks:

- Use a set of thin, colorful sticks.
- Practice picking up individual sticks without disturbing the others.
- This activity promotes precision and fine motor control.

3. Precision Drawing:

- Draw intricate patterns or shapes on paper using a fine-tip pen.

  - Focus on maintaining control and staying within the lines.

  - This exercise helps refine fine motor skills and hand control.

Incorporating these hand-eye coordination drills and fine motor skill exercises into your routine can be both enjoyable and beneficial for maintaining and enhancing these essential skills. Adjust the difficulty level based on your current abilities and gradually progress as you feel more confident in your coordination and fine motor control.

CHAPTER 6

Gait and Walking Exercises

Walking Techniques for Parkinson's:

1. Big Steps Walking:

- Take purposeful and exaggerated steps while walking.
- Focus on lifting your feet off the ground and swinging your arms.
- This technique helps improve stride length and prevents shuffling.

2. Cueing with a Metronome:

- Set a metronome to a rhythmic beat.
- Sync your steps with the metronome, emphasizing a steady and controlled pace.

- This auditory cueing can assist in maintaining a more regular walking pattern.

3. Visual Imagery Walking:

- Envision walking along a straight line or following a pattern on the ground.

- Concentrate on maintaining a straight trajectory, promoting better posture and balance.

- This technique engages both mental and physical aspects of walking.

Treadmill and Outdoor Walking Programs:

1. Interval Training on Treadmill:

- Incorporate intervals of varying speeds and inclines on a treadmill.

- Alternate between brisk walking and slower recovery periods.

- Interval training can enhance cardiovascular fitness and overall walking endurance.

2. Nature Walks:

- Walk in natural surroundings like parks or trails.

- The changing terrain and scenery provide additional sensory input, promoting a more engaging walking experience.

- Outdoor walks also offer fresh air and a connection with nature.

3. Social Walking Groups:

- Join a walking group in your community or online.

- Walking with others not only adds a social component but also provides motivation and support.

- Group walks can be organized in outdoor settings or on treadmills, depending on preferences.

These walking techniques and programs are designed to address specific needs related to Parkinson's while promoting physical activity and overall well-being. It's advisable to consult with healthcare professionals to determine the most suitable strategies based on individual circumstances.

CHAPTER 7

Speech and Swallowing Exercises

Articulation and Vocal Exercises:

1. Tongue Twisters:

- Practice tongue twisters to improve articulation and clarity.
- Start slowly and gradually increase speed.
- Examples include: "Peter Piper picked a peck of pickled peppers" or "She sells seashells by the seashore."

2. Pitch Variations:

- Work on varying your pitch while speaking.
- Practice going from high to low tones and vice versa.

- This exercise helps maintain vocal flexibility and expression.

3. Lip Trills:

- Gently blow air through closed lips while humming.

- Move up and down the musical scale with the lip trill.

- This exercise warms up the vocal cords and promotes control over pitch and tone.

Swallowing Techniques:

1. Chin Tucks:

   - Before swallowing, tuck your chin to your chest.
   - This helps close off the airway and may reduce the risk of aspiration.
   - Hold the chin tuck for a few seconds before swallowing.

2. Multiple Swallows:

   - Take small, manageable bites or sips.
   - After each swallow, wait a moment, then swallow again.
   - This technique aids in clearing the throat and minimizing the chance of food or liquid remaining in the mouth or throat.

3. Supraglottic Swallow:

   - Inhale deeply, then hold your breath.

- Swallow while holding your breath, followed by a strong cough.

- This technique can help protect the airway during swallowing.

These articulation and swallowing techniques are designed to enhance speech clarity and ensure safe swallowing. It's advisable to consult with a speech-language pathologist or healthcare professional to tailor these exercises to individual needs and address specific concerns.

CHAPTER 8

Relaxation and Stress Management

Breathing and Meditation Practices:

1. Deep Belly Breathing:

- Sit or lie down in a comfortable position.

- Inhale deeply through your nose, expanding your diaphragm.

- Exhale slowly through your mouth. Focus on making your breaths smooth and controlled.

- Repeat for several minutes, allowing your body to relax.

2. Mindful Meditation:

- Find a quiet space and sit comfortably.

- Focus on your breath or choose a calming mantra.

- Allow thoughts to come and go without judgment, gently redirecting your focus to your breath.

- Practice for 10-15 minutes to promote mental clarity and relaxation.

3. Guided Imagery:

- Close your eyes and imagine a peaceful scene, such as a beach or forest.

- Engage your senses by visualizing details like colors, sounds, and textures.

- Spend a few minutes immersed in this mental imagery to alleviate stress and induce relaxation.

Stress-Relief Strategies:

1. Progressive Muscle Relaxation (PMR):

- Start by tensing and then relaxing different muscle groups.

- Begin with your toes and work your way up to your head.

- This technique helps release physical tension and promotes overall relaxation.

2. Time Management Techniques:

- Break tasks into smaller, manageable parts.

- Prioritize important activities and set realistic goals.

- Effective time management can reduce stress by creating a sense of control and accomplishment.

3. Hobbies and Leisure Activities:

- Engage in activities you enjoy, such as reading, painting, or listening to music.

- Taking time for hobbies provides an opportunity to relax and shift focus away from stressors.

- Incorporate enjoyable activities into your routine to foster a sense of well-being.

Incorporating these breathing, meditation, and stress-relief strategies into your daily routine can contribute to a more relaxed and balanced life. Experiment with different techniques to find what works best for you, and consider seeking guidance from professionals if you need additional support in managing stress.

CHAPTER 9

Caregiver Support and Involvement

Exercises for Caregivers to Assist Patients:

1. Assisted Chair Squats:

- Stand behind the patient as they sit in a sturdy chair.

- Instruct them to stand up, providing support as needed.

- Guide them back down to the seated position.

- This exercise helps strengthen leg muscles and improves mobility.

2. Gait Training with Support:

- Assist the patient in walking, providing support if necessary.

- Focus on a steady and coordinated gait, encouraging proper heel-to-toe movement.

- Use assistive devices like walkers or canes if required for stability.

3. Seated Arm Exercises:

- Sit the patient comfortably in a chair.

- Hold their wrists or hands and guide them through gentle arm exercises.

- Include movements like lifting arms, rotating wrists, and reaching overhead.

- This promotes upper body strength and flexibility.

These caregiver-assisted exercises are designed to engage both the caregiver and the patient in physical activity, fostering a collaborative approach to maintaining mobility and overall well-being. Always consider the individual's capabilities and consult with healthcare professionals for personalized guidance.

CONCLUSION

In the world of managing Parkinson's disease, where each day can feel like an intricate dance with uncertainty, exercises tailored for this condition offer more than just physical movement. They become a beacon of hope, resilience, and newfound vitality.

Through the stories of individuals like Sarah, these exercises transcend the realm of mere physical routines. They become narratives of triumph over limitations, empowering individuals to navigate the challenges of Parkinson's with renewed strength and determination.

From gentle stretches that release the grip of rigidity to balance training that instills confidence, these exercises foster a sense of control and agency. Muscle strengthening, cardiovascular workouts, and coordination drills not only strengthen the body but also fortify the spirit, proving the resilience ingrained within.

Moreover, these exercises go beyond physical benefits. They enable individuals to reclaim the joy of movement, the freedom of expression, and the pleasure of everyday activities. They instill a sense of hope, fostering a community that supports and encourages each other through shared experiences and triumphs.

The guide to exercises for Parkinson's disease isn't just a manual; it's a transformative journey, a testament to the interconnectedness of physical and emotional well-being. It offers a pathway to a life lived with vitality, purpose, and joy.

As we close this chapter, it's not merely the end of exercises; it's the beginning of a narrative, a narrative where every movement signifies resilience, every step signifies strength, and every triumph signifies the indomitable human spirit. These exercises pave the way for a life filled with hope, possibility, and a vibrant celebration of the human capacity to thrive despite the challenges of Parkinson's disease.

FITNESS

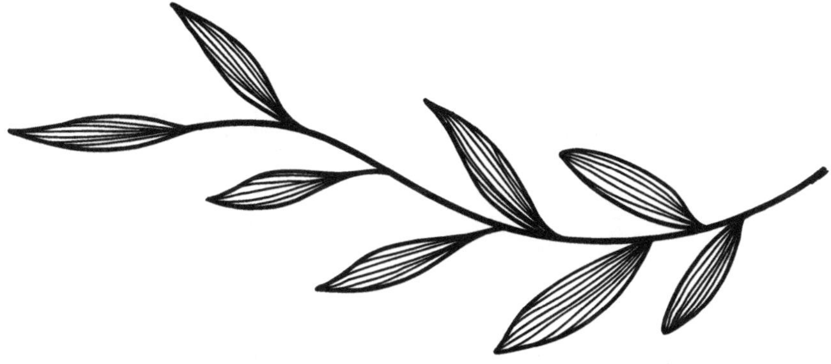

PLANNER

Fitness Planner

NAME: **DATE:**

BREAKFAST

LUNCH

DINNER

SNACK

EXERCISE

SET

REP

NOTES

Fitness Planner

NAME: **DATE:**

BREAKFAST

LUNCH

DINNER

SNACK

EXERCISE

SET   REP   NOTES

Fitness Planner

NAME: **DATE:**

BREAKFAST

LUNCH

DINNER

SNACK

EXERCISE

SET   REP   NOTES

Fitness Planner

NAME: **DATE:**

BREAKFAST

LUNCH

DINNER

SNACK

EXERCISE

SET   REP   NOTES

Fitness Planner

NAME:

DATE:

BREAKFAST

LUNCH

DINNER

SNACK

EXERCISE	SET	REP	NOTES

Fitness Planner

NAME: **DATE:**

BREAKFAST

LUNCH

DINNER

SNACK

EXERCISE   SET   REP   NOTES

Fitness Planner

NAME:

DATE:

BREAKFAST

LUNCH

DINNER

SNACK

EXERCISE

EXERCISE	SET	REP	NOTES

Fitness Planner

NAME: **DATE:**

BREAKFAST

LUNCH

DINNER

SNACK

EXERCISE **SET** **REP** **NOTES**

Fitness Planner

NAME: DATE:

BREAKFAST

LUNCH

DINNER

SNACK

EXERCISE

SET   REP   NOTES

Fitness Planner

NAME: **DATE:**

BREAKFAST

LUNCH

DINNER

SNACK

EXERCISE

SET   REP   NOTES